Chipmunka Anthology Volume Two

Introduction

Welcome to the Second Chipmunkapublishing anthology. We have decided to publish Chipmunkapublishing's shorter books in paperback so that we can give a voice to more people. It is our commitment to our authors that every Chipmunkapublishing title can end up having their work featured in paperback. Some of these books are quite short and would not be long enough to feature on their own as a paperback so putting several stories together enables books that may have only been e-books to come out as paperbacks. This anthology has 3 books inside it.

A Journey into Madness
Analgesia, Anna Last

Chipmunka Anthology Volume Two

A JOURNEY INTO MADNESS

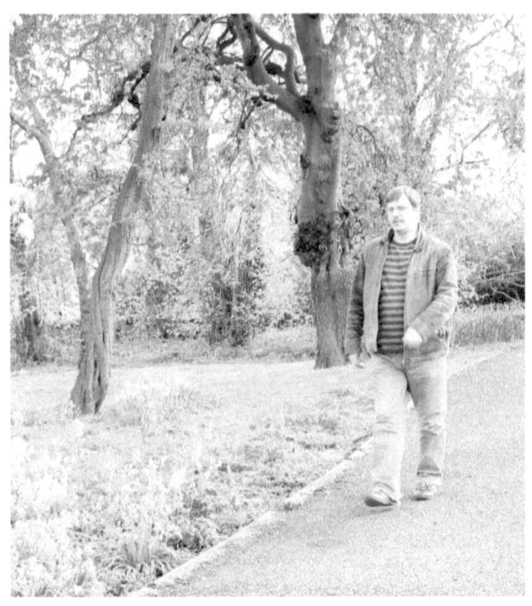

By Alistair McIntyre

'One million people commit suicide every year'
The World Health Organization

Published by
Chipmunkapublishing
PO Box 6872
Brentwood
Essex CM13 1ZT
United Kingdom

http://www.chipmunkapublishing.com

Edited by Mary Dow

A story of schizophrenia

Voices

I was working in Bedford in 1994 and decided to come home to Edinburgh. I had been feeling a bit paranoid and wanted to get back to familiar surroundings. So I decided to get a bus to Milton Keynes and from there home to Edinburgh. The bus from Bedford left at three o'clock in the afternoon so I got myself organised and made sure I was on it. Once I got to Milton Keynes I discovered there was a three hour wait until the bus left for Edinburgh, so I walked around the town wasting time. At 7:30pm I got on the bus for what I thought would be a 6 hour journey, but another journey was about to start which would last several years, a journey that was not expected but one that was to change my life forever.

It started as I was travelling from Milton Keynes to Edinburgh and had just crossed the border from England into Scotland. As the bus crossed the border I heard a voice shouting "shit, shit, piss, piss, fuck this". My first thoughts were that there was a disturbance on the bus. I stayed calm and just looked out of the window. More and more voices joined in "shit, shit, piss, piss". So I stood up and looked round the bus. To my surprise everybody was asleep. I didn't know quite what to think, but I could still hear these voices shouting.

After much consideration I came to the conclusion they were the voices of spirits. Yes, that was why they called Scotland God's Country, I reasoned, because people's spirits could speak to you. This must have been the case because it happened when I crossed the border, so the location must have had something to do with it. Everybody was asleep, nobody appeared to be shouting and nobody was being disturbed by the voices; it must be spirits. This shouting continued until the bus came into Edinburgh. Then everybody started making a noise as they got off the bus and the voices stopped. I got into a taxi, went to my mum's and went to bed.

The next day I was feeling a bit paranoid but decided to go out anyway. I walked from my mum's house in Granton to Newhaven, where I used to play as a child. I wandered all round my favourite childhood haunts: the adventure play ground, the old railway and the harbour. Then I went into one of the local pubs for a pint. As I sat down and started drinking my pint, I couldn't help notice that when people spoke to me they seemed very angry and aggressive. This wasn't how I remembered Newhaven. I decided to drink up and leave. As I walked home a man approached me and asked me the time. The way he spoke made me think he was helping to keep me under surveillance in order to inflict some harm on my person. It wasn't anything he said but a feeling I got when he spoke to me. This made me suspicious of everyone I met on the road back to my mum's house. All the way along the road my senses were very alert. I noticed the slightest movement or the faintest sound and was relieved when I reached my destination.

Later that night in my mum's house, when everyone had gone to bed, I felt a presence and assumed the spirits were back. So I lay on the floor to welcome them and hopefully listen to what they had to say, but there was only silence. After about two hours I went to get up when a voice shouted stay down. This was a scary voice and filled me with fear. Then loads of voices started shouting abusive things at me, calling me all sorts of names and accusing me of things I hadn't done. Then one voice shouted above the rest "gut him like a fish!" This made me jump to my feet terrified. A gentle voice then spoke and said "we're only trying to initiate you". I calmed down and lay on the floor again expecting to be initiated, but the voices just laughed. Then I went to my bed and fell asleep.

On the following day, Wednesday, I got up really early, after about three hours sleep. It was still dark outside. I decided to get dressed and go out. I had always enjoyed going round graveyards and reading the headstones and decided that was what I was going to do that day. I walked up to the cemetery at Crew Road, past the Western General Hospital. As soon as I had entered the gates I heard a familiar voice, that of a friend I hadn't seen in a long time; he clearly said "Do you want to play spirits?" I looked round and laughed. I didn't expect to see anybody there because by now I had come to recognize the difference between the voices of people who were there and the voices of spirits and this was definitely a spirit's voice. "Good one" I thought, to which the spirit answered "woooo". This I found very funny and I laughed aloud. I also realised I didn't need to talk to these spirits but could think things and they could hear me.

I started work the following Monday and everyday I heard more and more voices, sometimes they were friendly or funny and sometimes they were angry, accusing and frightening. The voices also became more frequent as the weeks went on. I then began to think I had been chosen by God to hear spiritual things. I began to have less and less to do with people and became more and more consumed with these spirits. People, I began to believe, were out to do me harm and they always seemed aggressive and threatening. The voices were also telling me that they were conspiring against me because they were jealous of my spiritual gift. I had begun to trust the voices; I had also learnt to fear others.

Visions

After working for about five weeks I had saved up enough money to pay for a bed-sit. I viewed several and eventually found one in a respectable and quiet house in Broughton Street. I thought immediately that I could be happy here, so I moved in right away.

I was still hearing voices but began to notice something else as I watched the television and listened to the radio. Sometimes the people on the television and radio would be speaking to me personally. This was a novelty at first and it got me quite excited. I couldn't believe it: the T.V. and radio giving me messages. These messages were pleasant at first but as the months passed they changed and left me feeling responsible for the disasters I heard about on the news programs. So I stopped watching television and listening to the radio and started going to the pub instead.

I remember speaking to people in the pub, mostly women as I found men to aggressive. I soon noticed that I could tell what they were about to say or do, as if I were psychic. I then realised that they could hear my thoughts as well. This was a bit scary but fascinating. So I experimented by thinking about particular people in the pub and saying things in my thoughts. To my amassment the people seemed to react to my thoughts which confirmed my belief that I was telepathic and psychic. The problem started when I tried to switch off. Some of my thoughts were nasty and the whole pub was hearing them. I started to become scared. Maybe someone would attack me or at best someone might be nasty or start shouting at me. So I decided to leave the pub and go home.

While walking up the road I started to calm down and relax again. When suddenly out of the corner of my eye I saw a light; this light appeared to flutter like a bird, it shot upwards and disappeared. I wondered what it was. Then a voice spoke saying "it's a soul", so I marvelled at seeing such a magnificent thing. Over the next few weeks I saw more and more souls quite often being accompanied by the voice of a spirit. One night I was walking up Leith Walk and it was nice and peaceful without much happening. I was having a great day. When suddenly out of the sky came a scream and a massive ball of light flew straight towards me, I ducked, it flew past and disappeared. A voice then spoke "that is all the souls of the people in Leith going to hell, tell them about Jesus." I felt guilty after this because I thought that I had helped condemn them.

A few days later I was watching people in the street from my bed-sit window. A particular man caught my eye. He had stopped at the bus stop and was reading the bus timetable, when all of a sudden his spirit stepped out of his body. I knew it was his spirit because it was exactly like him, same size and shape except it was transparent, I could see right through it. God has blessed me to see spiritual things as well as hear them I thought and my heart filled with joy.

I started seeing more spirits and souls as the months went by. The spirits started invading every part of my life, sometimes helping, sometimes inflicting pain on me and at times the souls and voices were tormenting me mentally. I couldn't watch T.V. or listen to the radio. I also felt responsible for the disasters on the front pages of the papers which filled me with guilt. I had a lot of periods at this time when I felt miserable but there were still moments of great joy. I was still working through all this. I didn't have much to do with my work mates though, apart from when I was warning them about hell and telling them about Jesus a result of one of my visions accompanied by voices.

Hospitalisation

After stopping listening to the radio, watching television and reading the papers, I found that I had a lot of time on my hands while in my bed-sit. So I decided to read text books on psychology. It was while I was reading one of these books I that found out about nerve endings. These give us our sense of feeling, allowing us to experience pleasure and pain. This discovery formed a question in my mind and I began to become obsessed with finding an answer. Who could I ask? I thought. Nobody I knew had any knowledge of psychology. I thought about going to a college or university but it was night time and they were closed. I needed an answer to my question and I could not wait until the morning. I had heard there were psychologists and another group of professionals with knowledge on the subject of psychology, psychiatrists, at the Royal Edinburgh Hospital, so I decided to go there that night. I walked from Broughton Street to the Royal Edinburgh Hospital in order to see a professional and obtain the answer to my question.

When I reached the hospital it was about 9p.m. and all the doors at the front of the building were closed. So I went round the side to Mackinnon House where there is an out of hours reception. There was someone on duty, a lady who said "Can I help you?" and I replied "Can I see a psychologist, as I have a question to ask them?"

To this she informed me that there were only duty psychiatrists there at the moment. So I asked to see a psychiatrist. The lady then asked for my name, to which I replied "Alistair McIntyre". She then disappeared after asking me to wait a moment. About five minutes later two people, one man and one woman, appeared at the door which led into the hospital and said "Could you come with us Alistair?" They led me into a small interview room where we all sat down round a square table. I was facing the door, the lady was on my left hand side and the man was facing me with his back to the door. They introduced themselves and asked me "What is the problem?" I answered "There is no problem, I have just got a question to ask". The man replied "What is the question?" "Well" I said "are sexual pleasure and physical pain automatically connected?" At this the male psychiatrist jumped to his feet, pushing the chair back with his legs, and cried out "What sort of a question is that to ask anybody?" I simply replied "It is just a question", while wondering why he was reacting in this way. The man then said "I would like you to come into hospital for a few days". I said "okay".

I could not help thinking, as I sat with the woman and the man went to make arrangements, that this must be a joke; after all I only came in to ask a question. The man then returned and we started making our way up to Ward 3. Once there I received a medical, where they took my blood, tested my reflexes and asked me a series of questions. I was then shown to my room, which was a private room on the right hand side as you came into the ward. It was at this point I thought, maybe they need the work and that is why they have asked me to stay in hospital for a few days. I also thought I will get a few days holiday from my work. So I went to join the people in the ward in the smoking room and tried to settle in for the night.

The people in the ward all left the smoking room at about 10p.m. and started queuing in the corridor for their medication. Once they had received their medication the nurse came looking for me and found me smoking a cigarette. She had two white tablets she wanted me to take. “What are they for?” I asked. “It’s what the doctor prescribed” she replied. “What are they? What side effects do they have?” I enquired. “The doctor said you were to take them.” She said. “I am not taking them, there is nothing wrong with me and I don’t know what they do.” I said. After half an hour of trying to persuade me to take the tablets she finally gave up and I went to bed. I couldn’t help thinking, while I was in bed: what do they think is wrong with me? Eventually I went to sleep.

In the morning I was woken up by another nurse offering me more tablets, which I again refused. I then got up and went to the smoking room for a cigarette. While having my cigarette I spoke to some of the patients and told them how I came to be there and how the staff kept trying to give me medication. I also told them how I was worried about the side effects and that it was strange them giving me medication when nothing was wrong with me. One of the patients, a young woman named Tracey, told me about a book called the BNF which listed all medication and side effects. She said she knew this because her step-father was a doctor. So I went into the office and asked to see a copy of the BNF. The staff asked me what I wanted it for, then refused to give me the book saying “it might get lost.” I explained that I wanted to see what the tablets they kept offering me did and what side effects they had but the only thing they told me was the tablets were called Chlorpromazine.

Later that day Tracey's step-father, John, came into the hospital to see her. He had with him a copy of the BNF, which he gave to Tracey, who then showed it to me. I looked up Chlorpromazine and was horrified when I saw the side effects; I was also shocked to read that this tablet was given to people who were psychotic. I couldn't believe it: here was I, only there to make up the numbers in order to keep the doctors in work, and they were trying to get me to take tablets with horrific side effects.

A few days went past and I had not taken any medication because of the side effects. By now I had had enough and thought: they can't keep me in here when there is nothing wrong with me. I had been repeatedly told: you won't get well if you don't take the tablets. So I decided to ask for a diagnosis. I went into the office when a lady psychiatrist was there and asked for one. She said "why do you want a diagnosis?" I explained that they could not hold me there without one. She then said "That's easy; you have schizophrenia." I could not believe it. So I decided to gather as much information as possible on schizophrenia. I disagreed with the psychiatrist after reading the information but could do nothing about it. So I felt trapped and helpless and realised the only way I was going to get out now was to take the tablets which I started to do.

Moving Wards

After being in hospital for five days and not seeing anybody I knew, I decided to call my mum. She came up to see me right away. When she arrived the psychiatrist asked if he could speak with her in private. After the interview, my mum told me she had told the psychiatrist I was homeless. She then persuaded me to give her the keys to my bed-sit in order to get clean cloths for me. My mum then left the hospital, went to my bed-sit and moved all my stuff out, leaving me homeless and in hospital. My mum's words to me were "you'll get a house out of it." The psychiatrist then decided, that as I wasn't resident in the catchment area for ward 3 but was homeless, I should be moved to the ward for the catchment area of my mum's address; ward 6. So I was moved to ward 6 and instead of having a private room I was given a bed in a dormitory.

After a few days of being in ward 6 I discovered, through my conversations with the other patients, that I could leave the hospital. So I went into the office and told the staff I was discharging myself. The staff said I would have to see a doctor first, so I agreed. About half an hour later a psychiatrist appeared and took me into a room. I told him I wanted to discharge myself and he asked me a few questions about my reasons why. After answering his questions he said "you can leave if you wish." So I left immediately. I went to my mum's house that night, because I had nowhere else to go. Because I had left the hospital in such a hurry I had left my personal belongings behind. I decided to pick my stuff up the following day.

So I went back into the ward the next day. The difference this time was that I felt in control. I went to my locker, emptied it and headed for the exit. When trying to leave one of the staff said “oh, you’re back in the ward.” “No, I’m just picking up my stuff and leaving” I replied. I was then told I would have to see a doctor first and reluctantly I had to agree. A couple of doctors then asked me a few questions. I was then led into a room with five people in it. A woman on my right hand side started reading a sheet of paper she had in her hand saying “You are being held under the Mental Health Act Section 26”, when I interrupted by saying “You can’t tell me that you can read that piece of paper and I can’t get out of here.” “Yes I can” she said and carried on reading. I couldn’t believe this, they were all serious. I was trapped, helpless and confused. The woman then finished reading, and then they opened the door, to take me back to the ward, when I saw my opportunity to escape. I was off and running, jumping down flights of stairs and tearing through corridors, being followed by a male nurse who was lagging behind. Out the side door, over the grass, straight up a stone wall and then I stopped dead. On the other side of the wall was a builder’s yard. I quickly reasoned that, if I went in that yard, I’d be charged by the police for trespassing. By now the nurse was at the bottom of the wall and said with an out of breath voice “Please come down”, so I did. I was taken back to the ward, the door was locked and I thought there is no chance of me getting out now.

While I was in ward 6, I met some interesting people and witnessed some strange, funny and scary events. The first person I got to know quite well was Samson. He was about 25. Quite a nice guy but had the strange habit of eating every plant that was in the ward. I remember when Samson and I were in the quiet room drawing and painting: Samson took a break. He sat in a chair next to a cheese plant and started eating it. I was a bit worried about this and said to him “That might be poisonous.” He just laughed and said “It tastes great, try some.” So I laughed and said “No thanks” and we then went back to drawing. By the time Samson got out of hospital he had eaten the whole cheese plant.

Then there was Roy. Roy was a bit of a loner. I remember one day he came into the dormitory when I was lying on top of my bed. He said “Hello” and went and lay on his bed. About five minutes later a nurse accompanied by a man entered the dormitory. The nurse asked Roy if he had taken a taxi from Glasgow and Roy said “Yes”. The nurse then said “You haven’t paid the taxi driver.” “I don’t need to, I’m mad” Roy said. The taxi driver, who was the man accompanying the nurse, then started shouting and saying he wasn’t leaving until he got paid. Roy refused to pay the man, continually saying “I’m mad.” The nurses started to gather round Roy and spent about an hour trying to persuade him to pay the taxi driver, which they eventually succeeded in doing.

A strange and frightening event that took place concerned a girl named Lucy. Lucy was a nice, friendly girl. We used to play cards while I was on my section. One day she was chatting away quite normally and we went into the corridor and sat down on the seats. We were in the corridor for a while, when suddenly she jumped to her feet, kicked in a window, fell to the floor and rolled about screaming “Get them off me.” The staff came running from all directions, grabbed her, held her still and gave her an injection by force. They moved her out the ward and I never saw her again.

After completing my section and three days of close observation (when I wasn’t allowed out the ward), to my delight I was released on pass for a few hours at a time. It was at this time that I was asked by Tracey (the girl who had given me a copy of the BNF) if I wanted to go to the bowling club. I remember thinking: I’m not travelling down to Granton from Morningside, where was the only bowling club I knew about. When Tracey found out that I thought the bowling club was in Granton, she informed me that there was one in the hospital grounds called the Tipperlin. Tracey and I spent a couple of hours a week in the Tipperlin Bowling Club, drinking lager. I was amazed that you were able to drink alcohol in the hospital grounds; I felt like this was a reward to the patients, for good behaviour and conforming to the hospital rules.

The Pass

After being in hospital for approximately two months, I still felt there was nothing wrong with me. I had been taking the medication and obeying all the rules. As a result, the time I was allowed out of the ward had increased from a couple of hours at a time to 9am to 9pm everyday. I took full advantage of this and only came back to the ward for food and medication at 12pm and 6pm. I felt I had to conform or be confined to the ward. It was around about this time that I was asked by the psychiatrist if I would like to go to my mum's house for the weekend on a pass. I jumped at the chance. Arrangements were made and I was about to have my first real taste of freedom for what seemed like a long time.

When I arrived at my mum's house, I thought I wouldn't have to take any tablets or obey any rules until I got back to the ward on the Sunday. My mum made sure I took my medication four times a day and I was in the house every evening, so I didn't get the freedom I expected. When everyone had gone to bed though I could do what I wanted, except leave the house. On the first night, at about 3 o'clock in the morning, I decided to make myself toast. I remember putting the bread on the grill, then suddenly feeling terrible and afraid so I crouched on the floor in the corner of the kitchen. I lost all track of time. The next thing I remember hearing was my step-dad shouting "fire, fire!" The toast had burst into flames and the smoke was belching out into the sitting room. Luckily he had gotten out of bed to go to the toilet, smelt the smoke and investigated it. The fire was put out and I was told to go to my bed, which I did.

The following day I decided to go up the town. I had heard there was an exhibition on at the National Gallery in Princess Street and told my mum I wanted to see the paintings on show. While this was true I also had another reason for going. I had painted a picture while in hospital on a large A3 peace of paper and wanted to show it to people at the exhibition because I thought it was an exceptional work of art. I got on a number 16 bus and headed for Princess Street.

When I arrived at the art gallery I was delighted to see it was busy. I went in and looked round the exhibition until I saw somebody who I thought looked like they knew a lot about art. I approached him and said "There's some really good paintings here, don't you agree?" I carried on "I'm a bit of an artist myself, in fact I've got one of my paintings here in my coat." The man then said "Can I see it?" "Certainly, I would value an opinion on it as I haven't shown it to anyone and I was thinking about exhibiting it," I said. I then took the large peace of paper I had rolled up out of my jacket and unrolled it. The man looked at it, looked at me and smiled. "What do you think?" I asked. "It's a mushroom, a big mushroom" he replied. "That's right, it's a Boletus Edulis or Cep" I said. The man then left and I went home to my mum's quite happy that the man knew what it was.

On the Sunday I decided to visit my brother, Robert, at his work, before going back to the ward. He was working in a hotel near Morningside. I arrived there at about 7pm. I wasn't feeling very good; I was hearing a lot of voices and seeing visions of spirits that were disturbing me. When I entered the bar I asked one of the staff if I could speak to Robert the chef and they said they would just fetch him. When he appeared we spoke for about five minutes and he bought me a pint. Robert then said he was very busy as it was dinner time and I was to take a seat and enjoy my pint. While I sat drinking my pint I got very confused. Everybody seemed to be talking all at once and I couldn't separate one conversation from another. Then a large Alsatian dog appeared and I watched as its spirit ate off everyone's plate, which I found very unhygienic. I then felt like the dog was going to bite me so I left without saying cheerio to my brother and went back to the ward.

Back In The Ward

A few days after my pass had finished, I was again getting used to life in the ward. Then Scott was brought in. He was a quiet guy, but used to stare a lot at me. Once he had been there a couple of days, he asked me if I had a spare cigarette. He said he would return the cigarette to me when his visitors came in to see him, so I gave him a cigarette. Half an hour later he asked me again. I didn't mind at first because I knew what it was like to go without one. However, this continued all week and I got fed up of supplying him with cigarettes and the visitors never came. So I bought him a packet of cigarette papers. I then took a paper from the packet and proceeded to make a roll up for myself from the dog ends in the ashtray (something that a lot of people did in hospital) and said to Scott "this is how you survive with no money". He looked at me a bit surprised, but made a roll up from the ashtray anyway. He continued to do this until he eventually got a visitor who brought him tobacco.

Another person who came into the ward was Helena. The only English words Helena could speak were Bosnian,coffee, good and yes. One day Tracey and I were in the quiet room when Helena came in. She smiled and said "Bosnian coffee" while beckoning us with her arm. So Tracey and I followed her and she led us to her room. In her room she had a flask, some small cups and sugar. She poured us a cup of Bosnian coffee from the flask and said "good, yes?" So we tasted the coffee and agreed it was good. We stayed in Helena's room for about two hours drinking Bosnian coffee, saying good and smiling at each other. I remember feeling like we had all had a very pleasant experience, even though we couldn't understand each other.

Someone else who came into the ward at this time was Paul. Paul and I had some great times talking to each other. I remember speaking to him about what he wanted to do with his life. He told me he wanted to be a clown. He also told me he had dressed up in a clown's outfit and had gone about the streets of Edinburgh making people laugh. He said he had enjoyed the experience so much that he had given up university, where he had been studying to be a lawyer. This had outraged his parents and as a result they had him put in hospital. Paul insisted there was nothing wrong with him and he was going to follow his dream and become a clown. So we had a good laugh about this, then I went for a cigarette.

When I went to bed that night I spoke to Paul again. He slept in the bed next to mine and a curtain separated us, which we pulled away. We chatted for hours. Then at about 3am a group of nurses came into the dormitory, passed my bed, surrounded Paul and pulled the curtain back into position. I now couldn't see Paul, but I heard him saying "What is it?" There was no answer. Then

Paul started screaming and went silent. I found out later that they had given him an injection to put him to sleep. The thought of this happening to me terrified me.

Another day on the ward, about a couple of weeks later, I was in the smoking room (as I was most of the time). It was quiet and I was enjoying my cigarette. It was nearly always quiet, before something happened. I suddenly heard someone moaning as though they were in pain. I ignored it at first, as did the nurses, but it continued. The moaning was coming from the corridor, so I went to investigate. I saw in the corridor something that shocked me. I found a woman, who had shit on the floor, and she was rolling around in it. Immediately I reported it to the staff. They then confined everybody to the smoking room, while they dealt with the situation. About an hour later we were allowed out the smoking room and things on the ward were back to normal.

Being Discharged

After being in the ward for what seemed like a very long time, I was starting to notice improvements in my mental health because of the medication. I was now able to recognize that I had a mental illness and that a lot of the things I had experienced were not real. The voices and visions had stopped, the delusions had gone and I was feeling pretty good about myself once again.

I was still having regular meetings with the psychiatrists, which I experienced all during my time in hospital. Now the psychiatrists had called a meeting which was to include my mum and step-dad. This meeting was to discuss my immediate future. The first thing I remember was, that instead of taking tablets, as I had been doing, the consultant psychiatrist said she would like me to go on an injection once a week. I said "No." Then my step-dad piped up and said "I think it would be better if you had an injection." The two psychiatrists then joined in and started giving me reasons why they thought an injection was the way to move forward. I began to feel pressured into going along with what was being suggested. As this trio of my step-dad and psychiatrists went on, I felt the pressure build up until I exploded. "No fucking way" I shouted. I then looked at my step-dad and said "You have an injection." The room went silent. After a couple of minutes one of the psychiatrists broke the silence and said "You will have to keep taking the tablets then." "For how long?" I enquired. I was told that I would have to take them for the rest of my life as there was no cure for schizophrenia; it could only be controlled by medication. The next thing I remember being discussed was where I was going to live. The psychiatrists wanted me to live in a hostel for people who had a mental illness. I refused point blank. I said "I'm going back to work when I get out of here and I'm not staying in a hostel." They seemed quite surprised at this and said "We'll have to change your medication then. Pimozide would be best as you only take one tablet a day, but the dosage won't be the equivalent to what you are taking now." I agreed to take this drug, the meeting ended and I went back to the ward.

The following day I was taken by a nurse downstairs to an examination room. When I was in this room a woman asked me to strip to the waist, which I did. She then placed these little sticky suckers, with wires coming out of them and connected to a machine, around the area of my chest where my heart is. When I asked what she was doing she said that this was a cardiograph and it was to see if my heart was healthy. I then asked why I needed a cardiograph and was informed that it was because of my new medication. I remember thinking: I won't be taking those tablets for long, not if I have to go through all this before I can take them. So the woman did the test and said my heart was healthy. I got dressed and left.

After the examination I went to the welfare office in the hospital where I had an appointment. I was sat down on a chair and it was explained to me that because I was homeless I would need to fill in an application for a council house. I was then asked the questions on the form and the woman filled in the answers for me. At the end of the interview I signed the form and she told me she would send it away and hopefully it wouldn't take too long to get a house. I thanked her and went back to the ward.

A few weeks later I asked the staff if I could go back to work. I was told I could. So I started going to work from the hospital. I would get up at 6 a.m. in the morning, have some cereal and wait on the door being opened so I could go to work. Coincidentally Tracey started going back to work from the hospital at the same time and we used to have a laugh while waiting in the corridor. It was at this time I was told that if I was working from the hospital I would have to pay for my board. However, I only did it for a week and was discharged at the weekend to my mum's house, so it didn't cost me anything.

I had stayed at my mum's house for approximately two weeks when a letter came through the door offering me a house. I was quite excited when I saw the letter but when I read the address of the house my heart sank. It was in a part of Leith that I knew was really rough. My mum said "You'll like, it having your own place", and I felt she was putting pressure on me to take the house. However, upon reading the letter again I discovered, to my delight, that the viewing date had passed and I had missed the house because the letter had come via the Royal Edinburgh Hospital. About another week later another letter came with another offer of a house. This time the viewing date was in a couple of days' time. The address was 80/5 Sleigh Drive. When I viewed it I thought: this is great, a lick of paint and a bit furniture and it will be perfect. I accepted it and as soon as I was given a moving in date I signed the lease and moved in.

So five and a half months after my hospital admission I was now free. The first thing I did with this new found freedom was cut off all connections with the medical profession. I stopped taking the tablets and felt my life was now my own, I was the one making the decisions, whether right or wrong it was my choice and I loved it.

The Next Year

In the following months I enjoyed my freedom to the fullest. I started seeing my friends again. We would sit in each others' houses in the evenings, chatting about the things guys talk about, generally having a laugh and listening to music. At the weekend we would go to the pub. Occasionally after having a few drinks in the pub we would go onto a club. Sometimes if I had a date, I would go for a meal and then to the pictures, but only if there was a good movie showing. I worked hard and played hard. Life was great and I thought my journey into madness was over.

Then about seven months after stopping the medication the voices started again. When this happened my immediate thoughts were, is this normal or is it part of an illness. I began to reason; this happens to everybody when they reach a certain age but no one talks about it, it is part of growing up. I did not seek any help because of this reasoning but decided to keep it under control. Keeping control was really easy at this stage. The next thing that started happening was I started sensing spirits all around me, until one day at my work, I noticed the spirits were controlling me. In fact I began to believe I could do nothing without them. Spirits had been controlling me all my life, I reasoned. Before I had been unconscious of this but now I had become awakened to this fact. I felt useless, like some spirits' puppet, but I carried on thinking I was normal.

As the months rolled on the voices and spirits became worse. The voices would tell me I was being poisoned by the spirits, which I believed, because I could see the spirits putting things in my food. I remember one time I was in my mum's house and she had made my dinner. It was chicken, mashed potatoes and sweet corn. I was late on arriving for dinner because I had worked a little late. So I sat in the dinning room alone. When I was given the plate of food I thanked my mum and she left. I then put my arms around the plate and bowed my head, covering the plate so the spirits couldn't put anything into it. I reasoned if I lift my hands and head to get the knife and fork the spirits will poison my food. In the past few days the spirits had thrown stuff into my food making it inedible. So I ate the food with my hands, like an animal. It was the first thing I had eaten in three days. I remember thinking, as I washed my hands, if you don't learn to control these spirits you will never be a complete adult. I then went through the living room and started telling my mum that the psychiatrists did not know what they had been talking about and that there was nothing wrong with me. She said "I could have told you that. If there had been anything wrong with you it would have shown when you were a child." This made me more determined to control the spirits and voices.

I still worked all day but instead of enjoying my evenings and weekends, I endured them alone in my flat. I had stopped seeing my friends and became pretty isolated and paranoid. People once again seemed aggressive and threatening. One experience I had confirming to me that all this was normal was when I was sitting in my living room. I could hear the voices of spirits in my head. These voices started kidding me on; then suddenly they became aggressive and threatening. I stood up and said "I'm not afraid of you lot." The voices then started saying they were going to beat me up. This continued for what seemed like ages. I then said angrily "Right - meet me in the stair." There was never anyone in my stair, so this would let me know for sure if the voices were normal or not. I opened my front door, walked along the corridor and started walking down the stair, where to my astonishment I met six men. I was determined to show no fear so I walked straight at them. They walked round me and said "Hi". I immediately calmed down and felt like I had won a great victory and thought it is defiantly true- the voices are real.

It was around this time I stopped sleeping. I would try and sleep but the voices and spirits kept me awake all night. I would work all day, come home and go to bed, then lie awake until the alarm went at six in the morning. This insomnia lasted for four days. I began to think I didn't need sleep; I had been wasting my time for years sleeping when I could have been doing things. On the fourth day without sleep my mum came up to the flat. She was going to wait in my house to let council workers in while I was at work. I told her I hadn't slept and she said I wasn't to go to work. Instead I was to go back to her house and she would call the doctor to see if he could give me something to help me sleep.

When I got to my mum's house I went to bed in the spare room. Almost immediately I fell asleep. I remember being woken up by my mum who told me to come through to the living room. My G.P. was sitting there and the first thing she said to me was "I would like you to go into hospital for a few days." I then said "What you mean is if I don't go you'll have me sectioned." She said "Yes." So I agreed to go, the ambulance came and I was once again in hospital, approximately five months after the voices had started again and one year after my discharge.

Hospital again

Once in hospital I was placed in ward 3, the ward for my catchment area. On arrival in the ward I was given a medical. During this medical the staff took blood samples and the psychiatrist asked me several questions. It was during this interview that I was asked if I would take part in some tests the hospital was doing on a tablet called sulparide. It was explained to me that this was an anti-psychotic medication, and if I agreed to take part in this experiment I would be given 200 milligrams four times a day. I was also informed that I would be monitored to see if there were any side effects. So I agreed to take part in the test. I was then asked how many siblings I had and if any of them had problems with their mental health. I told the psychiatrist about my brother Ian who had had a mental breakdown but was doing fine now. I was also asked if I thought my immediate family, of brothers, sisters, mum and dad, would agree to have a blood test. The reason I was given was that the psychiatrists were trying to see if there was a connection between schizophrenia and genes. I told the psychiatrist he would have to ask my family if they would take part in these tests, which he agreed to do. The interview ended and I went back to the smoking room in the ward.

The following day my mum and sister, Carol-Ann, came up to visit me. While they were there the psychiatrist asked them if they would allow him to take a blood sample, explaining to the two of them about the tests they were doing. My mum and sister said, “If it helps Alistair we will.” They were then taken away into a room where blood was taken. My mum then organised for Linda, my other sister, and my two brothers to come up and give blood, which they did. However, we were never told the results of this research. After my mum and sister had given blood we all went to the Verandah Club. The Verandah Club is a café in the hospital grounds. On the way there my sister was walking behind me. This caused me to become paranoid and anxious. I remember thinking that she had a gun, which she had gotten from her husband who was in the army, and was pointing it at my back. So I started demanding that she walk in front of me, which she eventually did. This made me feel a lot more secure. When we arrived at the Verandah Club, I ordered a coffee, which was quite enjoyable. We then went back to the ward and my mum and sister left.

About a week later I was asked to go to the welfare office in the hospital. So I went down and was informed that my employer had terminated my contract and I had to claim benefits. The welfare officer then filled in the appropriate forms for me and sent them off. This left me feeling a bit depressed.

After I had been in hospital for about a month my dad came up to see me. I remember it well; he brought me cigarettes and rather than sit on a seat in the smoking room he turned the empty bucket upside down and sat on it. He then smoked a cigarette and put it out on the tiled floor. I thought to myself when he did this; he thinks he is at his work. He was a painter and sat on tins at his work like we all did. I told him about losing my job. As usual in situations like this he was able to cheer me up with one of his stories.

That evening after my dad had left I went to the Tipperlin Bowling Club for a pint. While I was sitting in the Club I heard a voice say “Hello stranger”, I looked up and saw Tracey. She said she had been bored and had popped in to see if she knew anyone. We chatted away all night, catching up on what had happened over the last year. She then asked me if I wanted to go back to her flat, which I did. When I arrived at Tracey’s flat I phoned the hospital ward. I told them I was staying with a friend that night and I would see them tomorrow. They told me that I couldn’t do that and was to come back to the ward, so I said “See you tomorrow” and hung up the phone. I hadn’t told them where I was staying in case the police came round looking for me and took me back to the ward. We had a good laugh about the nurses’ reaction on the phone. When I went back to the ward the following day nothing was said to me.

A couple of days later I was interviewed by a student psychiatrist. She asked me if I was feeling depressed or sad: A question I always answered

"No" to. The reason for this was that I knew one of the treatments for depression was electro-convulsive therapy (E.C.T.). The very thought of receiving electric shocks through my brain terrified me. She then asked me if I became very happy. I said, "Not really, I'm quite stable with my mood." Then she asked me a question nobody else had asked, "Do you hear voices?" On hearing this I thought for a while, then said "I'll answer your question if you answer one of mine first?" She then enquired "What is your question?" "Do you hear voices?" I asked. She quickly replied, "I asked you first." The interview quickly broke down after that and I went back to the smoking room for a cigarette.

Approximately 6 weeks after I had been admitted the voices had stopped but instead of feeling great like the first time in hospital I was feeling pretty down. I had lost my job, was feeling a little depressed and my confidence had gone. It was at this time I was told I was going to be discharged. However, I was also told I would have to attend a day unit twice a week as part of my ongoing treatment. This unit was situated just outside the hospital grounds. So I agreed to go there as part of my treatment, then went home.

The Following Years

Once released, I attended the day unit faithfully for two months. During this time I was appointed a key worker. I always felt like the key worker was always pressurising me into doing things I didn't want to do. One activity I did enjoy though was the photography group. A group of us from the day unit used to go round places like the Royal Botanical Gardens, taking photographs. The following week we would develop the photos in a dark room; it was quite good fun. I soon got bored of the constant pressure to do activities in the day unit and eventually stopped going.

The side effects from my new medication also got me down. I couldn't sit still, my legs kept bouncing up and down and people kept commenting on it. So I stopped taking the tablets and it wasn't long before the voices were back.

However, it wasn't all doom and gloom. Tracey moved into the area, just a few streets from where I was living. Before long we were going out with each other. We would sit in our houses chatting. It was Tracey who encouraged me to seek the help of a psychiatrist, as I told her I was hearing voices. So I went along to Inchkeith House where I saw a psychiatrist, who prescribed me the tablet Respiridone. My concentration during this time was very poor. I couldn't even read a short letter without having a feeling of despair. I couldn't remember to take my tablets, so the voices got worse. Then I started seeing visions. This was all too much for me, so I told Tracey and she told me to contact the psychiatric emergency team at the Royal Edinburgh Hospital, which I did.

I was again admitted into hospital. Only this time I was placed in Ward 1, as Ward 3 was full. I remember asking one of the staff in Ward 1 whether your spirit could leave your body while you were alive. She said "Your spirit could only leave your body if you were dead." I wasn't convinced by her answer as I felt like someone had stolen my spirit. The good thing about this admission into hospital was that within two weeks, I was discharged. I did, however, have to attend Inchkeith House, where I was given a community psychiatric nurse. This nurse would meet with me once a week, to see how I was progressing. I wouldn't say much during these meetings, only that I was doing fine and still taking the medication.

A couple of years later I married Tracey. A friend took us to a place called the Castle Group. This was a drop-in service for people with mental health problems. One of the good things about it was that it wasn't connected to the health service. I had lost a lot of my social skills, but attending the Castle Group helped me regain these, as well as restore my confidence. I only went to the Castle Group for about eight months before it closed.

A new-drop in was opened in its place called Safehaven. I played a big part in starting this group up; by going to meetings with the social work department, people from the health service, the voluntary sector and representatives from the Consultation and Advocacy Promotion Services (CAPS). I now attend the existing Advisory Management Group for Safehaven, as a service user representative. Because of this involvement I was asked to join the CAPS management committee, an offer which I accepted. CAPS is an organization that empowers mental health service users to have a voice in the planning of mental health services. It is a great privilege to play a small part in this organization.

My mental health is quite good now. I still hear voices occasionally when I'm stressed. I take my tablets regularly, increasing them myself if I feel I'm becoming unwell. I have a much greater control over my mental illness than I thought possible. It took me years to get to this point in my journey into madness, but the future is looking bright. I'm a grandfather and I have a good, stable, loving relationship with my wife, Tracey. I have made many good friends at Safehaven. I also have the support of my family and friends.

Analgesia
A Collection of Poems

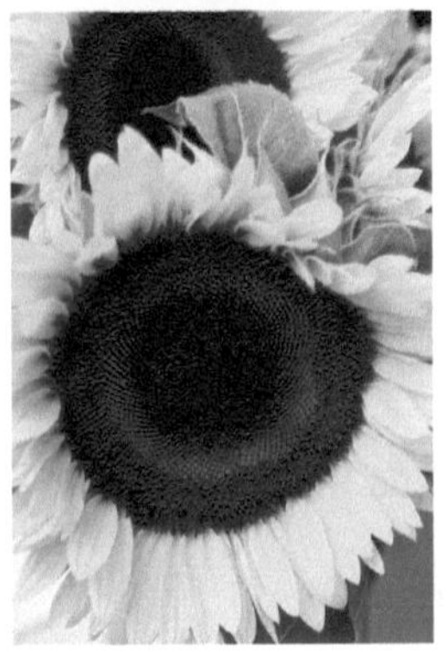

By Anna J Last

‘One million people commit suicide every year’
The World Health Organization

Published by:
Chipmunkapublishing
PO Box 6872
Brentwood
Essex
CM13 1ZT
United Kingdom

http://www.chipmunkapublishing.com

Proof-read by Sofia Ribereiro

CONTENTS

Volume I

Part One: Early Years 2000

Part Two: Malady 2000 – 2002

- - - - -

Part Two: Ditto 2004

Part Three: Let Out 2004

ANALGESIA

VOLUME

1

Preface

I began to express myself creatively from a young age, when communicating verbally became more and more difficult. As my confidence in communication declined, expression of feelings and emotions on paper became a preference. I never sat down purposely to write; instead writing offered me the comfort and attention that no human could offer. The page became my mentor in times of loneliness and despair.

The journey within these pages conveys my memories and experiences of life battling against clinical depression and Anorexia Nervosa. *Analgesia* became an escape from living, writing to erode the pain.

About the Author

Anna Last was born in Ipswich in 1977 and has lived on the Suffolk Coast for most of her life. In 1998 Anna gained a BA (Hons) in Geography from University of Hull and in 2001 an MA in Library and Information Studies from University College London. *Analgesia* is her first collection of poetry.

PART ONE:

EARLY YEARS

2000

The Search

Lost, I'm falling, lost I fall,
Do I really know where I am at all?
Lost, I'm searching, lost I ask,
Why is it so hard to leave the past?

Mind and brain, brain and mind,
Looking carefully what will I find?
An answer I must find if I can,
To establish who I really am.

Another Susanna Kaysen?
I too express myself through pen.
Another Esther Greenwood?
I would change if only I could.

Falling, searching, searching, fall,
Does anybody really listen when I call?
Help me, help me, let me take,
Before it's all much too late.

Un/ Control

Christmas is close,
The fear is nigh.
Control, stubborn, weak,
Greed, wanting, disgust.

Expansion, expansion, clothes,
Feeling tight against flesh.
Secrecy, guilt, vomit,
Sleep, exercise, anger.

Stabbing, abundance of weakness
Counting, much too much.
Overflowing shops, avoidance,
Stupid, battle, burn money.

"No thank you," maybe later,
Tables, people, stares.
Obsession, good, fruit,
February forgotten, Easter remembered.

Control high, control low,
Equilibrium, where?
Rotten, teeth fall out,
Exploding skin flying.

My Malady

The malady creeps through my body,
Crawling through every bone.
Swimming through my veins,
Heavy in my stomach like a stone.

The parasite lives inside me,
Controlling my brain and mind.
Dominating, other times lying low.
Is it my friend or foe?

Without my malady I could be alive,
With my malady I hardly survive.
Go away, leave me be,
The malady and me.

Fantasy Friend

Well,
My candle in the dark was not lit.
You never came today.
I waited, you never arrived.
I guessed you would not.
Disappointed.

Fallen,

My hurting heart aching.
It was for the best I know.
I warned myself,
Yesterday not to get excited.

Months will pass, before we meet,
Again.

Friend

Sitting here alone with just the rain,
I take your photo out again.
Your smile so comforting, I don't know why,
Embarrassed I look away and sigh.

Where am I with you right now?
It's gone on so long, I'm not sure how.
I am not yours and you are not mine.
Never really together all of this time.

Yet life without you, I don't know.
It's time to leave, I will go.
A fantasy, memory of the past.
We both knew it could never last.

So I know I have to move on.
Life must continue when you've gone.
I look once more, then put you away,
Into the box, to cherish, another day.

Truth

It's not what I think,
But what I feel.
Thinking is fantasy,
Feeling is real.

Almost

A gentle breeze blows through my hair,
Alive again I feel.

My delicate lips taste of salty sea air,

Alive again I feel.

Soft spring sunshine warms my cheek,
Alive again I feel.

The grey North Sea laps at my feet,

Alive again I feel.

Perfect white clouds dominate blue sky,

Alive again I feel.

Overhead gulls drift skilfully by,

Alive again I feel.

Pure white swans in salt marsh,

Alive again I feel.

Powerful light dazzles Marram Grass,

Alive again I feel.

For I know I'm leaving my cave behind,

As I recognise the beauty of the coast.

The erosion of loneliness I need to find,

Acceptance, love and care I search the most.

The Tube

Rats nibble on apple core,
Rubbish on the track.
Echoey shoes tap the floor,
Where bags are uniformly sat.

A rumble in the distance,
The rats all disappear.
Crisp packets begin to dance,
Moving closer, I have no fear.

Thundering rumble getting near,
Two headlights I can see.
A breeze blows my hair, so free.

The platform no longer clear.

Screaming brakes fill the air,
I stand on the yellow line, high.
The opportunity is very nigh,

I no longer have a care.

A jump and oh success.
A push and an arrest.
But too many people looking on,
All wondering why I have gone.

Library

Millions of documents live in my mind.
Looking carefully a variety to find.
Predominately they are archive,

Yet many currents still alive.

Classified by date,
Far more items than The Tate.
The older, the further back,
So many I often lose track.

The archives now delicate,
Should stay in their home at the back.
Carefully handling, so fragile,
Regularly slipping forward for a while.

Yet currents items are all that matters,
Otherwise retrospect become tatters.
Not all are found, yet I know they are there.
One day I will evaluate with great care.

Right now I must learn to concentrate,

On current documents before too late.
Leave the dusty archives be.
Look ahead, new documents I see.

PART TWO:

MALADY

2000 - 2002

Twisted

Twisting,
Knots and bones.
Plaits and veins.
Ropes and thoughts,
Twisting.
Raspberry ripple.
Weaved basket.
Pony's tail,
Twisting.
Inside,
My mind.

Pain

Like Versuvius lying dormant,
I lay in my bed.
Waiting for the time.
Years of energy to shed.

Commence eruption,
I scream and cry.
Flowing memories,
Of years gone by.

Back

Returning evil get out of my head.
Creature let me be,
Free from domineering darkness,
Creeping through my body.

Nature

Calmly, smoothly, I listen to her breathing.
Womanly, motherly, caring I feel.
The rise and fall of her chest, where,

My head rests, a baby against warmth.

Hurting

Place your arms around, my body
Fragile, delicate
Bones hold this torso
Together.
Embraced with me.

Wipe my tears away, from me
You take the pain, hurt,
Is lost, is hidden.
Safe in your arms.

Twins

Twins,
Anor and Rexia.
Twins,
Anor, known as Anna:
Good, happy, sane.
Twins,
Rexia, known as Rex:
Bad, sad, mad.
Twins,
Anna and Rex battle it out:
"Eat," "Don't eat." "Live," "Die."
Twins,
Anna and Rex,
Living in my head.
- - - - -

Why don't I rest my head?

Think of someone else instead.

She will never be mine, whatever I feel.

She is just fantasy Anna, not real.

I can not sleep, morning is far.
She is out there somewhere, a distant star.
She is all I think about,
Oh I must let these feelings out.

I want you, need you, so profound.

My feelings so sincere, so sound.
Defrost my mind, let the feelings melt,

It's hard to describe how my heart has felt.

Anatomy

One rests upon my clavicles,

The others live below.
Protection from the flesh supposed,

Yet peeping through mine show.

Hate

Shut up you nuisance,
I heard you the fist time.
Growling, grumbling within.
Please accept that,
YOU WILL NOT BE FED.

Aargh…

Aargh…aargh… steel stabbing sharp.
Pain heart hurt inside.
Knife indiscriminately plunges,
Stabbing, screaming, stealing…

Bath

With Ajax poured I begin to rub,
The cloth against the shiny tub
Obsessively wiping every bit,
This task feels like an endless pit.
I clean so hard, my knuckles sore,
God! I'm turning in to such a bore.
Fuck you" I scream, the dust won't go.
There are germs still hiding here I know
Compulsively, perfection, pushes me on
Cleaning while wondering where life has gone.

PART THREE:

OLDER

2002

Zopiclone

Zopiclone…
Swims down with water.
Zopiclone…
Night's panacea.
Zopiclone…
Drifting away…
Zombie Clone.

Analgesia

Analgesia, my panacea,
Erode this pain away.
Hurting, aching, abort it all.
Archive those memories,
Numb the past.

Precipitation

Rain hit's the roof with such force.

So heavy that it almost hurts.

I sit, held, let the tears flow.
Symbolically the intensity increases, to
Loud, powerful splats upon the window.
I have so much energy inside.
Just like today's weather
Stillness, event, silence, gone… only until,
Another day when I pour it all out.

Surrogate

"My nurse, my psychiatrist, my therapist…"
Pepper conversations like currents in a bun.

Dominate thoughts and decisions.
Replacement of reality, synthetic fantasy.
So intimate, yet impersonal,
Assembly line attention.
A prescription for living,
A prescription for dying.
A substitute for love?
Fills the empty gap of friends and family.
Cause denial of real love and support.
Yet professional surrogacy keeps me alive.

Nursey

Nice nursey, why do you nurture?

Is it in your nature to nurture?
Why are you so nursey nurse?
Nice by nature not nasty.

What is Love?

Impossibility of love, to love.
Not now, never.
Irrational desires to try it anyway.
End up hurt, confused, numb.
Re-enforces impossibility for love,
Enduring desire to try it again.

Fluid

Warm burning fluid trickles on,
The silver sharp sterile blade.
Trenches open divided…

Little Girl

She sits alone in the corner of the room,
Curled up small.
Little, delicate she feels.
Five years old again.
Tiny torso, flat chested,
Girly long straight hair

Unnamed

He pushes hard, hurting in.
Good? Ha! More bad.
Lying still, must,
Concentrate.
Better move, awkward.
Hurry up, faster, impatient.
Thoughts miles away.
Over, relief,
Humiliation.

Paranoia

It's always been there watching.
Like God looking down on Christians.
I don't know who or what, or even why.
Yet I know it is this that I must please.

This is what hands out punishment
It causes guilt.
A faceless creature always right.
I wish it dead.

ANAESTHESIA

VOLUME
2

PART ONE:

DETAINED 2003

ECT

I get in the taxi, my nurse in tow,
Check my name bracelet and off we go.
Across the road to the treatment suit,
Hungry I feel, nothing to drink nor eat.
Notes handed in, wait in a shabby room,
I know I'll be called in very soon.

Off with my shoes, I climb on the bed,
Wires attached to my chest and head.
"It's best not to look" the nurse advises me,
As I watch the anaesitist put a canula in me.
Inquisitively staring at the canula in my limb,
Brace myself for painful anaesthesia injected in.
Sweet smelling warm pain creeps up my arm fast,
Yet I can't speak as they place on an oxygen mask.
A strange smell and taste I can't identify,
My eyes flicker badly, unconsciousness nigh.
Seconds later I give up the sleepy fight,
Oblivious for a few minutes, then back to light.

Slowly I wake from synthetic sleep,
Don't want to move feel strange and weak.
Forced from bed to sit in a chair,
I wobble as my nurse helps me there.
Tea and a biscuit I have to consume,
But nausea, my head spins around the room.
All I want is to be home in my bed,
To stop this nausea and rest my head.

Taking forever, the taxi is here,
Wish he'd drive quickly, my vomiting fear.
I lie on my bed for the rest of the day,
Knowing tomorrow morning I'll feel okay.

E

Frying sausage sizzled in a pan,

Electric chair for a murderous man.

Burn alive along tender nerves,

Powerful machine with wired curves.
Jolted shocks executed,
Shaking hot body electrocuted.
Wavered flashing green and blue,
Dazzling light bulb blindingly new.

Shocks

Zip zap,
Electric crap.
Erode the cell,
That makes life hell.

Seclusion

In this cell it feels like hell.
There're watching from the door,
Lying on the bare mattress on the floor.

"Let me out" I scream and shout.
I've done nothing wrong,

Punching walls, feeling strong.

Suddenly they no longer ignore,
Three men are in, pin me to the floor.
Cut wrists from air vent on the wall.

They're wearing gloves, I cry in pain.
As neck and wrists forward bent,
Waiting as the doctor is sent.

Female nurse from next door
Lorazapam jabbed in buttock skilfully,
As I'm crushed face down painfully.

A duvet later arrives.
Along with Zopiclone,
Tonight this cell is my home.

Morning light, I'd slept the night,
Confused, dream or real fright?
Door open wide, quiet, get out.

Escape

Sick and sectioned I try to escape,
Once made it as far as the hospital gate.
Stand by Foxhall Road in bare feet,
Dark, quiet Sunday evening street.

Watching occasional cars pass by,
Realising their impact not enough to die.
As I wait fir a heavy lorry to come along,
Four hands grab my shoulders, back to where I belong.

Numerous occasions I've tried to run,
Once my absence noticed they will come.
On radios I hear it announced,
Make it across the field, then they pounce.
Strong male nurses catch me and restrain,
Kicking and shouting taken back again.
Here I am observed like a hawk,
Ready to try again when staff are short.

Specialled

Every moment, every breath,
With me to prevent my death.

Watching,
Sitting, at the door.

Watching,

Observing, 7-24.

Every minute, every hour,
Watching,

Looking while I bath and shower.
Watching,
Toilet, period, take a peep,

Dressing, watching while asleep.

Sectioned

I don't understand why they're done this again,
Used the Mental Health Act to detain.
I am not crazy, nor mad,
I've done nothing wrong or bad.
I'm just feeling a little unwell,
Suppose life has become hell.

But I don't need a psychiatric ward,
Alone, humiliated, confused, bored.
No matter how much I scream and shout,
Try to escape, they won't let me out.
Confined here in this prison like cell,
Two doctors, a social worker have made this hell.

Charcoal

"You need to drink this, it won't be nice."
Why sympathy when I'm paying the price?
Vomit bowl given, "You'll probably be sick."
Plastic bottle poured out to drink very quick.
Chalky blackboards dance in front of my face,
Down it at once, don't stop, so I can't taste.
McDonalds strawberry milkshake, smooth coal soap,
This slippery concoction sliding down my throat.
Pleased it's all gone, it wasn't so bad,
Yet if they think I'm drinking the rest they're mad.
Child's story of a wolf with a chalk softened voice,
Harder to drink the rest, but I have little choice.

Dye left around my lips like sucking a Black Jack,
Heavy stomach full of swimming antidote black.

Olanzapine

Overdose with packet of tablets stored,
Life too much again, collapsed on the ward.
Ambulance arrives, rushed to A & E,
No memories of this or them undressing me.
Zopiclone like experience, twenty hours of sleep,
Accident and **e**mergency ward I awake, weak.
Paralysed and speechless, confused and drowsy,
Invaded by monitors wired to my body.
Nearly died, rescued in time, failed death,
Experience disappointment, determined to take my last breath.

Ocean Eyes

Oh, though deep blue ocean eyes,
Meeting you was such a surprise.
I never knew I could feel like this,
Especially when so sick and helpless.

Oh, those deep blue ocean eyes,
A complex personality in disguise.
Chemistry between us when we touch,
Never felt this way about a man so much.

Oh, those deep blue ocean eyes,
Love at first sight I began to realise.
Hours spent laughing, playing chess, walking,
Every opportunity together talking.

Oh, those deep blue ocean eyes,
Made me tingle, heart beat rise.
Different background, I didn't care,
Missed you days when you weren't there.

Lindsey 1

Early morning light,
Sitting in the court yard.
Wearing just pyjamas,
Lindsey had taken me out.
She lights a cigarette,
Surprised I say "I'm shocked
To see you smoke - you're a nurse."
She laughs "Do as I say,
Not as I do sweetie."

Lindsey 2

It's only a few nights a week,
That Lindsey is here.
Out of place,
Too posh for the NHS.
Small and curvy,
Mothering.
Always cropped trousers,
Blonde hair tied up.
Long pointy straight nose.
I enjoy talking with her,
She lives near me.
Always tucks me into bed,
And rubs my hand goodnight.

Calories

It may have wiped my memory,
Of recent weeks and months generally.
Vague memories of my Italian holiday,
Forgetting events from August to May.

Yet ECT helped my obsessed mind,
When I search for facts I can not find.
Eroded memorised numbers and weights,
Fears of crisps, chocolate and cakes.

For Anorexia the best treatment I've had,
Although never cured my feeling sad.
For nearly a year I could eat again,
Around food, I suddenly felt sane.

Prolonged Summer

Heat wave hot summer, July to September,
Hottest October that I can remember.
Long, hot sunny days spent outside,
Thinking autumn will never arrive.
Body tanned from hours in the sun,
Being taken for walks was fun.

PART TWO:

DITTO

2004

Search

Pillows lifted,
Sheets shifted.
Mattress inspected,
Cupboards explored.

No pins or knife,
Nothing to risk life.
Allowed to bed,
Protected head.

Chance

Accidental mistake,
Noticed nearly too late.
A life probably lost,
A job certainly lost.

I chose to ignore,
Your medicine bag on my floor.
Darkness, under the chair,
Confused, why was it there?

Purposely left for me to use?
A test to see if I would choose?
No, you were totally unaware,
Fallen from your bag under the chair.

A decision I had to make,
Desperate, I just wanted to take.
Selfish, I couldn't do that to you,
After everything you had helped me through.

Staff Nurse P

You just sat and held me on the bath,

You did not shout, judge or laugh.
Pools of red on the bathroom floor,
Legs, arms and neck terribly sore.

I let you in so you could see,
What was about to happen to me.
Sharp glass bottle by the basin side,
Shower noose hanging where I had tried.

Back in my room you put me to bed,
Tucked me in, duvet pulled to my head.
A hug goodnight, your cheek touched mine,
Almost a kiss, but you remembered in time.

Bag Puss

We stuffed you in the clinic,
Cotton wool balls we put in it.
We fragranced you in my room,
With lavender oil perfume.

Zipped up to preserve the aroma,
To help with this awful melancholia.

My shiny bead bracelet we made in red,
Kept safely inside you while I'm in bed.

A pencil case in disguise,
Your arrival was such a surprise.
Pink and white stripy soft coat,
Warm and relaxing to stoke.

A nurtured gift for me to keep,
To calm me at night and help me sleep.
A substitute for human care,
To hug when alone and nobody there.

Alone

Away from the twenty-four hour hustle and bustle,
With only golfers and trees that rustle.
A picnic bench to rest and watch,
The golfers attempt another shot.

Peace and quiet, with nobody near,
Alone to think, get my head clear.
I see an old rubber tyre, could tie to a tree,
To use as a noose, but a golfer might see.

A shiny used bottle sparkles in the grass,
I smash it to create pieces of sharp glass.
Save it for later when back on the ward,
To use when suicidal, hurting or bored.

Mandy

Words can not describe,

How you helped me to survive.
Not knowing how I felt inside,
Your care kept me alive.
Your presence gave my mood a lift,
Only at weekends you did night shift.

Hugs

She gave me what I wanted,
What no one else would give.
She read my mind, knew what I needed,
Without my having to ask.

Others had tried, giving only a little,
Teasing, leaving, left wanting more.
But what you gave was so much,
Genuine, un-clinical care.

You rubbed my arm for half an hour,
And many times more.
Regularly you held my hand,
Remembering my hug each night.

"You pretty girl" she told me,
Always calling me "darling"
"They don't know what they're missing out,"
A game of ask and tell.

Dawn

It's 6am and already light,
I wake thinking it's still night.
Creeping passed the office empty,
I try outside door handles gently.
Amazed, unexpectedly both doors unlocked,
Escape again, my path unblocked.
In pyjamas and socks on dewy grass,
Don't look at the windows as I pass.
Confused, drugged, don't know where to go,
Early shift workers see me, so
Taken back to the ward where I belong,
Night staff not even aware that I'd gone.

Nightfall

Again nightfall arrives fast,
Anxieties of time spent here in the past.
Wandering men throughout the night,
Into my room, giving me a fright.
Protect myself as nobody else will,

Vulnerable once given the pill.

Wedge my door shut with a chair,

Fire regulations, but they don't seem to care.

Duvet and sheet pulled tight to my head

Full length pyjamas I wear in bed.
Bedside lamp on all night,
15 minute checks to see if I'm all right.
Vivid memories disguised in a dream,
Wander into lounge, no staff to be seen.
Alone and unsafe, I hide in my room,
Longing for morning to arrive soon,

Greatest Gifts of All

Tesco's sparkling orange water,
Mugs of steaming hot milk.
Sharing of Digestives and Malteasers
A plate of three jam sandwiches.
Sparkling beads and threads to use,
A Bag Puss pencil case.
A pack of tissues when mine ran out,
Promised garden bluebells but I'd gone.

All such special gifts I did not expect,
Yet nothing compares to your time and hugs,
Conversations, laughs and trust.
It's true that best things in life are free.
I owe you so much, Mandy.

Attachment

"You've become too attached to a nurse,"
Oh no, not again, this curse.
Debbie, then Kim, Julie and Sally,
Angela and Angie, Lindsey and Mandy.

Ethics and boundaries, always in the way,

Professionalism and codes of conduct stay.
Nurses are not friends, whatever I feel,
All in my head, fantasy, not real.

Trial

It's them against me,
Judge and jury.
Doctors decide my fate,
My life is on stake.
Consultant absent,
SHO lent.
Yet not sure who's side,
My nurse and CPN reside.
So it's them versus me,
Should I be set free?

Have my section removed?

Case must be proved.

Solicitor does job well,
Tries to remove me from hell.
Two hours and they've reached a verdict
It's exactly what I had predict.
My turn to testify
That I have a right to choose to die
I have lost my case,
So am detained in this place.
They've removed my right to die,
Distraught, I can not even cry.

A Friendly Face

A friendly face,
In this place.
A nurse from the past,

Who calls me Miss Last.

He is nosey, but nice,

Giving me his advice

He knows I'm not mad,
Just feeling sad.

Asks questions that others don't dare
Ward joker, but he does truly care.
Treats me as an equal human,
Down to earth, funny man.

His friendly face,
A relief in this place.
Doesn't judge my past,
Makes me laugh.

PART THREE:

LET OUT

2004

Gill

How lucky I was to get you as my CPN.
I didn't know how great you were back then.
For years you kept my head above water,
Saved me from this depressive slaughter.
A god, a tourniquet, life saver.
Accepted, not criticised my behaviour.
A positive adult to look up to,
You stuck by me through and through.
Trust through truthful dedication,
Offering positive hope and determination.
Then, suddenly you were gone.
Confused, what had I done wrong?

A change of job, you could still be my nurse?
Continue to help with this anorexic curse.
Yet discharged from the eating disorder team,
Despite very ill s I've ever been.
I don't understand why you think I'm well,
Eating and depression makes life hell.
So there must be another hidden reason why.
It angered and upset me so much I cry.

So another CPN allocated to me.
"Experienced," they said, yet I was soon to see.
In terms of anorexia she hasn't a clue,
No experience or knowledge of this like you.
The situation I do understand,
Yet emotionally I still need your hand.
So alone I battle, still very ill.
While remembering everything you taught me Gill.

Doctors

Psychiatric doctors, a breed of their own.
Think they're superior up there on their throne.
The majority are foreign, Asian and African,
They are rarely a woman, usually a man.
English is good, yet accents strong,
Language a barrier, this is so wrong.
Good communicators psychiatrists should be,
Yet frustratingly they don't seem to understand me.
All except Kathy, tall and thin.
Serious, no smile as she always rushes in.
Brief case in hand, glasses on face,
Appears to understand about my case.
I like her, feel equal and not below.
No emotions she owns, they never show.
Yet it is the foreign men I always have to see,
In ties and suits they patronise me.

Hamster

A happy hamster,
Is a busy hamster,
Rummaging through its cage.

A busy hamster,
Is an inquisitive hamster,
Swinging from its cage.

Rosie

Rosie, Posey, sweetie,
Wakes, comes out to meet me.
Grapes and lettuce treat,
Brazil nut once a week.

Rosie, Posey, messy,
Eats a lot but fussy.
Paws clean her little face,
Snuggled in her sleeping space.

All You Need To Know About...

A series of “All You Need To Know About” books,
Range in titles from “Cats” to “Achieving New Looks.”
Useful guides with all you need to know,
Diagrams, facts, coloured photos to show.

Titles found in the library or book store,
About cooking and baking, cars and much more.
Placed amongst the section for hobbies and leisure,
To read and study for one’s own pleasure.

An essential guide when a hobby is new,
Concise books that will see you through.
Endless advice that never runs out,
All you need to know about.....

Inside Out

Meaningful mosaic of mixed media messages.
Exhibited expertly examples of expression.
Shared skills with similar statements, yet
Specific sense of singular subjects.
Achievements of arts accomplished, with
Gathered genius of generous guidance.
Evidence of enthusiasm and energetic emotions.
Success of self.

Wanted

All I ever wanted was for someone to be around,
Even though I looked it wasn't to be found.
All I ever wanted was for someone to show they care,
Even though I searched, I found nobody there.
All I ever wanted was for someone to hold me tight,
To comfort me and be there in the night.
But all I really wanted was unconditional love,
To have that special relationship I know I'll never have.

Secrets

All the years of pain bottled up inside,
Life stopped long ago when part of me died.
I told no one through fear and pride,
The feelings I had constantly denied.
It was on my own where I had cried,

Which is why the hurting is still deep inside.

www.ingramcontent.com/pod-product-compliance
Ingram Content Group UK Ltd.
Pitfield, Milton Keynes, MK11 3LW, UK
UKHW040010200726
13854UKWH00001B/130

9 781847 473820